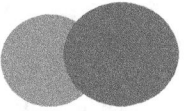

Table of Contents

Introduction

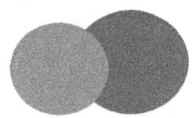

"The age of a woman doesn't mean a thing. The Best tunes are played by the oldest fiddles."
~ Ralph Waldo Emerson

Women in America have an average lifespan of 77.3 years, which is almost eight years longer than is seen in men. The projected population of US women in the year 2025 is 33.4 million versus 22.4 million men.

A lot of Gerontological research focuses on women. This is because the health and social problems of the elderly are increasingly those of women because their life expectancy is longer.

Following menopause, all women experience similar vulnerabilities as a result of age.

Some of the main vulnerabilities include physical and emotional manifestations of menopause, depression, and osteoporosis. Heart disease is the #1 killer of American woman, and most deaths are preventable.

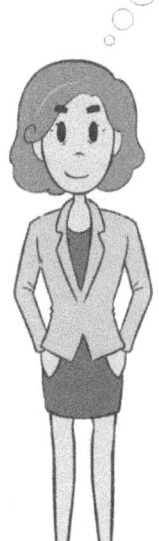

Quality of life into old age is of main concern for many, in maintaining optimal wellness and avoiding disabilities that threaten independence and the side effects of losing independent living abilities.

Many aspects of aging and its health related concerns require a thoughtful approach on the part of the woman in taking care of herself to promote the best possible life in older years.

Normal Aging In Women

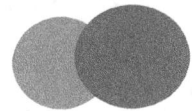

Certain things occur as the natural process of the passage of time, as the body begins to manifest age.

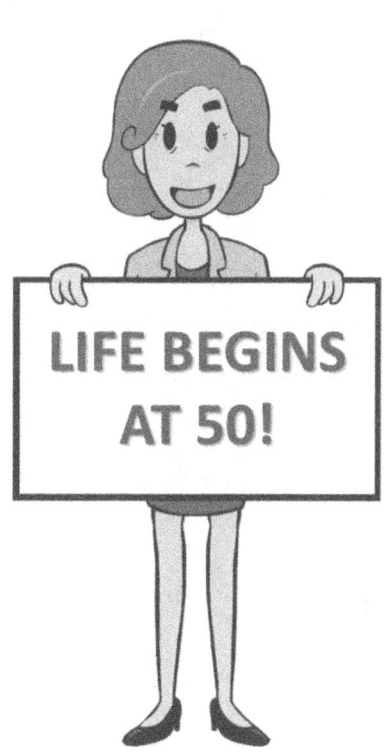

- Brain structure changes with age, many of the effects are still unclear to science, but older people do notice changes, including impact on memory.
- Heart muscle thickens, and arteries stiffen with age. This results in the heart having more difficulty pumping oxygen rich blood throughout the body and taking oxygen from the blood.
- Hearing naturally diminishes with age.
- Aging results in the body producing less hormones that control functioning of organs and tissues, including estrogen and growth hormone. More research is being conducted into this area of aging to understand its impact and to possibly counteract its effects.
- Immune system cells become less active with age, making humans more vulnerable to infection from viruses and bacteria. Researchers believe that this process may play a significant role in the overall aging process.
- The ability to breathe air in and out of the lungs decreases with age, which can result in shortness of breath while doing brisk activities.
- With age, the kidneys ability to remove waste from the bloodstream declines.
- An aging bladder becomes less able to hold as much urine.

- Older people lose muscle mass, and strength as they age. Women who do not engage in muscle building workouts will see a decline of up to 22% between the ages of 33 and 70. Late in life body weight declines and fat shifts from just beneath the skin to deeper organs.
- Aging skin thins and loses it elasticity that causes sags and wrinkles. Dry skin is seen in older women as a result of the loss of oil glands. Years of sum damage can cause spots.
- Hair becomes gray and brittle. Some women experience hair loss or thinning.
- Bone loss speeds up after menopause causing them to weaken and become brittle, which can lead to osteoporosis and increased risk of falls that can lead to injury and injury-related death.
- Eyesight diminishes in midlife, contributing to the booming reading glasses industry. Glare interferes with vision, and seeing well in low light situations becomes more problematic after the age of 50. Seeing detail can become a problem at age 70 and older.

Common Health Conditions In Older Women

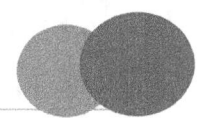

"There is a fountain of youth: it is your mind, your talents, the creativity you bring to your life and the lives of people you love. When you learn to tap this source, you will truly have defeated age."
~ Sophia Loren

As age catches up, women are vulnerable to certain medical conditions:

- Asthma is commonly diagnosed in older adults.
- Risk for cancer goes up with age, and especially breast, lung and colorectal cancer in women.
- COPD or chronic obstructive pulmonary disease is the 4th leading cause of death in the US and World, typically it is caused by smoking.
- The risk of diabetes increases with age and complications include conditions of the eyes, kidneys, nerves, and higher risk for heart disease.
- Heart Disease is the #1 killer of women, and most heart attacks are preventable.
- High blood pressure risk increases after menopause and women often experience no symptoms.
- Incontinence is very common among older women; statistically it affects 4 out of 5 women though it is not considered to be part of "normal aging."
- Chronic pain because of conditions such as arthritis, or fibromyalgia is common and pain can lead to depression.
- Stroke is common in older women and they die from stroke more than men do.
- Depression is common in older adults, but twice as many have it than men. Women whose husbands have died or those with a chronic illness are at a higher risk.

- Osteoarthritis is an age related condition that occurs when tissue that buffers and cushions the ends of the bones wears away.
- Balance problems are often caused by various medical conditions, disturbances in the inner ear and certain medications increasing the risk for fall.
- Dry skin is common as women age.
- Eyesight degrades through the aging process, most people over the age of 40 need reading glasses. For some, dry eyes or teary eyes also occur.
- Hearing loss is also often seen in older age.
- Some type of sexual dysfunction is reported by 1/2 of all women of senior or even middle age years.
- Insomnia and other sleep problems are more common with age.

Lifestyle Choices And Prevention

"At age 20, we worry about what others think of us. At age 40, we don't care what they think of us. At age 60, we discover they haven't been thinking of us at all." ~ Ann Landers

Prevention of disease in women is more than just taking prescribed pills and seeing your doctor regularly. You can naturally prevent disease through lifestyle changes that can improve your overall health without drugs and without doctor's visits. This doesn't mean you have to skip those things, however. It may mean, though, that you can avoid chronic illnesses, as you get older. It may also mean that you can age better, and live longer.

An ounce of prevention truly is worth a thousand cures, especially when it comes to heart disease, the #1 killer of women where most deaths are considered preventable.

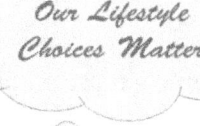

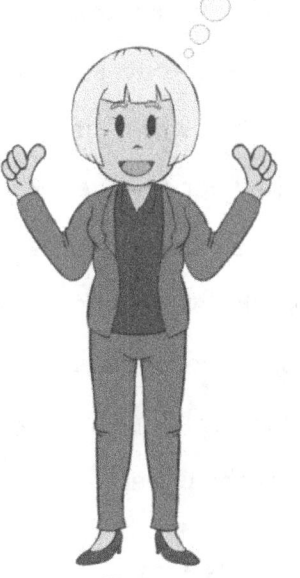

Tools To Prevent Disease

Many lifestyle choices can prevent disease if you stick with them.

Exercise

It has been repeatedly shown through research that prevention of illnesses can be accomplished through regular exercise.

What Kind Of Exercise Is Important To Consider?

There are two kinds of exercise that a woman can do to prevent chronic illness. These are aerobic exercise and anaerobic exercises.

Aerobic exercise involves any type of low, medium, or high impact exercise that gets the body moving so that you can reach a target heart rate throughout your exercise program. In aerobic exercise, you get your heart rate going and generally move your arms and/or legs vigorously enough to raise the heart rate. Examples of aerobic exercise include swimming, tennis, running, brisk walking, dancing, and cycling. Each has its advantages and disadvantages when it comes to the aging woman. For example, swimming is low impact so it protects the joints but it doesn't burn as many calories as, say, that running does, which is much higher in impact. You get to decide how much impact your muscles, ligaments and joints can handle.

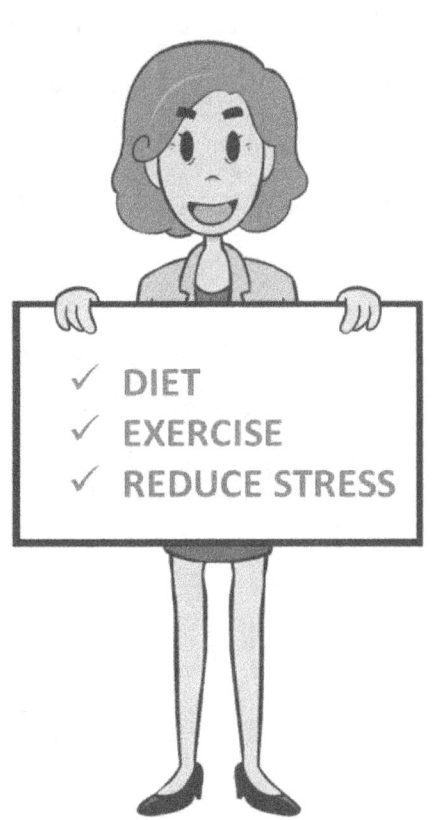

Anaerobic exercise involves weight lifting. You can use machines for lifting weights or just lift free weights. These workouts strengthen, tone, and build lean muscle mass, which increases the number of calories burned per day even when the body is at rest and helps in weight loss because muscle tissue is what burns calories. Whenever fat is replaced by muscle, you look leaner as well. Anaerobic exercise also protects your bones from osteoporosis because it strengthens the bones.

Which Exercise Is Best

Experts recommend *at least* 30 minutes or more of aerobic exercise five days a week and 2 or more days of strength training. If you only plan to exercise five days a week, then do three days of aerobic exercise and two days of anaerobic exercise.

Many American diets are nutrient poor and calorie rich. We eat far too much meat and processed junk food that contains trans-fats, which are used as a preservative for processed foods that must sit on a store shelf before purchasing. Cooking in oil, such as deep fat frying also means you are getting too much fat. You can begin your healthy diet plan by avoiding these types of foods and by eating foods that are higher in complex carbohydrates, and healthy proteins and fats.

A plant-based diet is rich in nutrients, low fat, low calories, and high in vitamins. They contain mostly complex carbohydrates that can help reduce sugar fluctuations in the bloodstream, which can lead to type 2 diabetes. They are also high in fiber, which lowers cholesterol, and helps bowel movements be less constipating.

Good Things To Eat In This Type Of Preventative Health Diet Include:

- Whole Fruits
- Vegetables
- Whole Grains Like Whole Wheat, Oats, Barley, And Rye
- Low Fat Dairy Products
- Lean Meats, Fish And Poultry

Whole fruits and vegetables contain antioxidants, which fight off diseases related to oxygen free radicals in the system, which are natural products of metabolism that require antioxidants to relieve the body of them.

Americans do not get nearly enough fiber in their diets and the recommended intake is:

- 25 grams for women younger than age 51
- 21 grams per day for women ages 50 and older

Fiber is found in whole fruits and vegetables. Juices of fruits, for example, often contain less fiber and only raise the glucose levels, leading to peaks and valleys in glucose that contributes to obesity because of elevated levels of insulin in your body during the peaks in sugar. When the insulin level has to rise because of a high level of sugar, it must put away the excess sugar as fat. Select foods with a low glycemic index, which means they do not cause spikes in blood sugar.

Maintain A Normal Weight

You need to maintain a normal weight while trying to prevent disease. Obesity and even lower than accepted weight levels can contribute to disease as women age. Obesity, in particular, can increase the risk of metabolic syndrome, heart disease and some weight-related cancers, like breast cancer and colon cancer. You can help yourself maintain a healthy and normal weight by practicing healthy eating and exercise habits. You will also look better and increase your level of self-esteem.

What Is A Normal Weight?

A normal weight is having a body mass index of between 19 and 25 (as long as you aren't a body builder with lots of heavy muscle on you). You can calculate your body mass index or BMI by taking your weight in pounds and dividing it by your height in inches squared, multiplying this number by 703.

A BMI between 25 and 30 indicates that you are overweight and a BMI of 30 or more means you are obese. Calculate your BMI and you might be surprised as the amount of weight you need to lose.

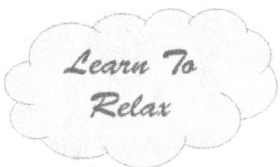

Reduce Stress

Stress reduction can be accomplished through lessening the amount of stress in your life and by practicing stress reducing techniques. Stress reduction can reduce your risk of stress-related diseases and can prolong your life.

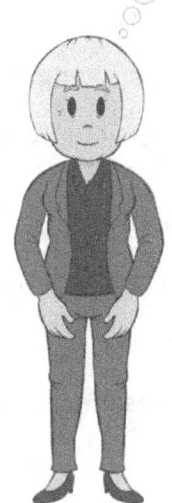

You can lower the amount of stress in your life and thus remain healthier by deciding which things in your life are the most stressful and eliminating them or modifying them.

- ✓ For example, if your job is stressful, think about talking to your boss or switching jobs altogether. If your relationship is stressful, contemplate relationship counseling or even personal therapy.
- ✓ You can practice stress reduction at home using meditation or ancient Asian health practices for stress reduction, including tai chi and qi gong. Yoga is another lifesaver.
  1) Meditation involves finding quiet place to sit or lie down while you close your eyes and focus on deep and even breathing, relaxing the muscles as much as you can. Meditation can involve using a special syllable or 'mantra' to bring you to a state of relaxation or visualization, which involves imagining yourself in a peaceful and beautiful place, like a garden or beach. The visualization of the sights, sounds, and smells of the place you come up with can relax your brain and body, leading to improved levels of the stress hormone, cortisol, so you don't suffer from stress related diseases.
  2) Tai chi and qigong can help you gain balance, grace, and a better state of mind through the practice of various movements tied into breathing and structured meditation. Both tai chi and qi gong have been linked to healing from specific diseases and the prevention of chronic illness. These are easy health practices that can be modified for those with less physical activity or who are bound to a wheelchair or bed.

3) Yoga can reduce stress, tone muscles and increase flexibility. You can practice yoga as part of stress reduction as well as a good form of exercise. Take a local yoga class or purchase a yoga DVD to learn the different poses and breathing techniques in the comfort of your living room.

Stress reduction, weight loss, eating healthy and exercise sound like simple ways of preventing disease and improving the aging process, but they really work and you can reap the benefits right away. As you lose weight and gain strength, you can fight off chronic illnesses like diabetes, heart disease, and obesity.

Other Key Methods

Seek Mental Health Services If Necessary

If you find yourself getting depressed or having problems at home or work, you can prevent a total meltdown, a psychiatric admission, or job failure if you seek preventative advice from a trained therapist. Through therapy, you can work with your spouse on improving your relationship, you can undergo family therapy, or you can seek individual support for any stress-related or emotional symptoms you have before they get too serious.

Stay Social

If you continue or newly develop a good social support, you will be sick less and will live longer than those who isolate themselves from others. Social support systems can help alleviate depression and can help you maintain good mental health and brain activity. Research has shown that those women with good support systems live longer and healthier lives when compared to women who didn't have good support systems.

Keep Close Family Relationships

If you have a family that has drifted apart, attempting and succeeding at bringing them together for family reunions and holidays can improve mental and physical health. It, like social interaction, has been shown to improve longevity and can give you a positive outlook on life. Getting in touch with your grandchildren as you, age can be a good way

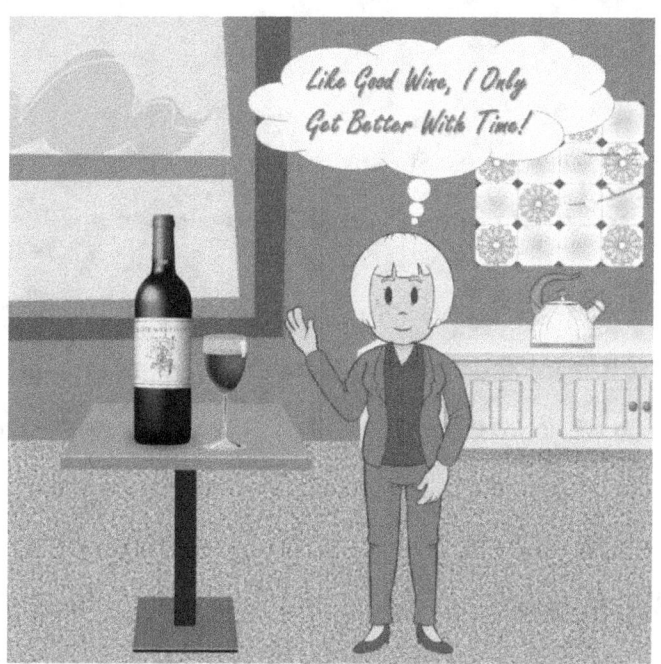

to feel young and recognize your value to these children as they age, too. This close family tie can bring about a sense of purpose as you teach your grandchildren and children the values in life that you learned as a child.

Quit Drinking

Alcohol can be consumed in limited quantities but not drinking any alcohol can be especially good for your health. For women, it is recommended that one alcoholic beverage per night is adequate but nothing more than that. Alcoholism is prevalent in older women, especially those that are isolated and have few family contacts.

Quit Smoking

It is never too late to quit smoking. Smoking can lead to lung cancer, heart disease, certain other cancers, and COPD. These days, smoking cessation programs are easier than ever and there are many medications besides nicotine replacement therapy that can help the smoker stop smoking for good. Many of the negative effects of smoking can reverse themselves after just a few years of smoking cessation.

Avoid Illicit Drugs

Drugs of any kind, even prescription drugs, can have side effects that include an early death from complications. This is especially true of illicit drugs, which have no benefit or healthy consequences. Staying drug free from drugs like cocaine, heroin, or even marijuana can contribute to better health and a longer life.

The trick to preventing disease and living a longer life is to isolate those things you are doing that are counterintuitive to good health and gradually lessen these habits in your life. You don't have to do everything all at once. Seek the advice of a physician or therapist when it comes to prioritizing the things you should do that will promote good health and prevent disease in your future life. Tackle one problem at a time and try not to procrastinate. Your health is important to you and you should take it seriously, especially as you age and your body can no longer handle the psychic and physical stressors you place upon it.

Preventative Medical Care

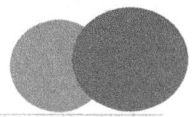

In modern medicine, there is an increase in focus on prevention of disease rather than on treating already existing diseases. What a concept! For this reason, as we age we need to focus on things that can prevent us from developing the typical diseases of aging, such as cancer, cardiovascular disease, and dementia. Lifestyle choices are just method to this end.

Women live an average of eight years longer than men live and need to do what they can to make these older years as healthy as possible. Here are some things a woman can do to improve her chances of living healthy as she ages:

Screenings For Physical Diseases

This includes seeing the doctor for various screening tests recommended for women of advancing age. For example:

Colonoscopy

A colonoscopy is recommended for both men and women beginning at the age of 50. This test is repeated every year to look for colon polyps, which can be removed before they become cancerous.

Stool

Stool for blood is checked annually and some women will have a flexible sigmoidoscopy at the 55-year and 65-year mark, in between colonoscopies.

Blood Sugar

Women should be screened periodically for diabetes, which tends to increase with age and with increasing weight.

Heart Health Checks

Blood tests to check cholesterol levels and other heart health checkups are highly recommended. Going over your family history and personal risk factors as to heart disease with your doctor can help with early intervention, as heart disease is the #1 killer of women.

Cancer Screenings

Cervical Cancer

Cervical cancer or cancer of the cervix is usually caused by the human papillomavirus (HPV), a common virus passed through sexual contact.

According to the American Cancer Society, cervical cancer was once one of the most common causes of cancer death for American women, though this rate has dropped 50% in the last thirty years as a result of Pap smear testing, which is a screening that tests for changes in the cervix before cancer develops. This allows for early detection when the cancer is curable.

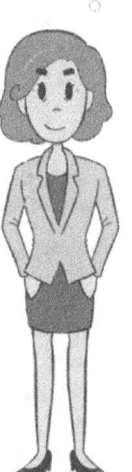

It's Never Too Late To Start Making Healthy Choices

Cervical cancer tends to occur in midlife and most cases occur in women younger 50. However, older women are still at risk as they age, and more than 15% of all cases occur in women over the age of 65, but they rarely occur in women who have regular screening tests before the age of 65.

- New screening guidelines set by the United States Preventive Services Task Force and the American Cancer Society now advocate testing every three years for women ages 21 to 65 as opposed to the previously used yearly tests. Screenings are no longer recommended for women under 21 years of age.
- 5 year screening intervals are recommended for women ages 30 to 65 when both Pap smear and Human Papillomavirus testing is done.

Breast Cancer

Breast cancer risk increases with age, according to the National Cancer Institute here are the probabilities of women developing breast cancer based on age:

- At the age of 40, the probability of development of an invasive form of breast cancer in the next 10 years is 1 in 69.
- At the age of 50, the probability of development of an invasive form of breast cancer in the next 10 years is 1 in 43.
- At the age of 60, the probability of development of an invasive form of breast cancer in the next 10 years is 1 in 29.
- At the age of 70, the probability of development of an invasive form of breast cancer in the next 10 years is 1 in 26.

Your individual breast cancer risk may be lower or higher, depending on but not limited to genetics, excessive alcohol use, family history, race and lifestyle habits.

Mammograms

A mammogram is an X-ray picture of the breast and this screening is recommended to test for early signs of breast cancer. As of today, this is the best test medicine has for early detection that can save lives.

- The United States Preventive Services Task Force recommends that women ages 50 to 74 have a mammogram every two years. Depending your family history, your doctor may recommend that you have mammograms before the age of 50 or more often than usual.

Self breast exams are recommended and notifying your doctor of any changes in the breast is another way to promote early detection.

Screenings For Depression

Many women suffer from preventable depression due to diseases like hypothyroidism. Low thyroid conditions can mimic depression and it is perfectly preventable. The screening test is a blood test and, if the test is abnormal, thyroid hormone can be replaced, correcting the fatigue, constipation, and memory impairment/depression seen in hypothyroidism.

Screenings For Dementia

Women should have a mini mental status examination at the age of 65 or older. If evidence of dementia exists, preventable causes of dementia can be looked for and treated.

If there is no prevention for the source of dementia, there are medications that can at least prevent the progression of the disease to some degree. Low thyroid conditions can mimic dementia and can easily be checked for using a simple blood test.

Bone Health

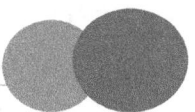

"I look forward to being older, when what you look like becomes less and less an issue, and what you are is the point." ~ Susan Sarandon

Women are at risk for osteopenia and osteoporosis more so than men are. They are relatively protected against bone loss because of the estrogen in their bodies but, when they reach menopause, the bone protection is lost and women begin to lose bone mass rapidly. It is said that prevention of osteoporosis is a lifelong battle and that those women with low bone density at age 20 will have a greater risk of developing osteoporosis by age 50-60.

There are several ways women can prevent bone loss or build backbone. Some represent lifestyle changes, while others are medications.

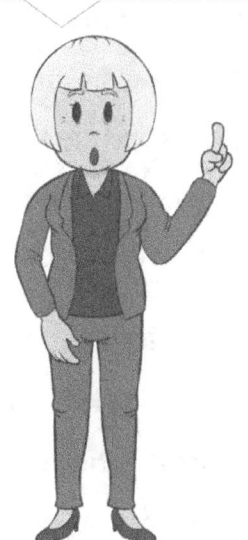

OSTEOPOROSIS CAN BE PREVENTED

Preventing Osteoporosis

✓ **Exercise:** Women who exercise will strengthen bone to prevent bone loss and fractures. The best exercises are those that involve mild to moderate impact, such as aerobics, walking, cycling, or dancing. These cause your bones to respond to the need for increased mass by making stronger bone. Exercise should ideally be a lifelong habit but it is never too late to start an exercise program for better bone health.

✓ **Calcium and Vitamin D:** Both calcium and vitamin D support bone health and deficiencies in either one of these nutrients can result in slow bone growth or in loss of bone that is difficult to replace. Vitamin D supplements and calcium supplements can be used to treat or prevent bone loss. The amount of vitamin D and calcium you need to take depends upon your age, the degree of bone loss you have already sustained and the type of calcium you take in. Certainly, you can't go wrong with milk that has been fortified with vitamin D. The milk has calcium in it and the vitamin D is necessary for the calcium to be absorbed and taken up by the bone tissue.

✓ **Eat yogurt:** Yogurt has many healthy constituents, not the least of which is that it is rich in calcium. Not all yogurts are fortified with vitamin D so you may have to take a vitamin D supplement in place of a food source of vitamin D and calcium together.

✓ **Take medications to build backbone:** Once you have already lost bone, it is difficult to get it back using an increased intake of calcium and vitamin D, even when using supplements. For this reason, medications are recommended by doctors. Some medications used for the treatment of osteoporosis include bisphosphonates, such as alendronate. This is a generic drug costing about $40-$60 per month. It has been demonstrated through research studies to prevent hip, spine and wrist fractures in those with documented osteoporosis by building up bone tissue and adding calcium to bone. There are many different bisphosphonates that you can use, some of which are oral, while others are parenteral shots taken every few months up to once per year. Many of these medications have side effects and are very expensive to take, even with health insurance. Alendronate is also called Fosamax, while other bisphosphonates include ibandronate (Boniva), risedronate (Actonel) and zoledronic acid (Reclast).

Talk to your doctor about whether or not you are at risk for osteoporosis. Women who are small-boned or are of Asian and Caucasian descent are at a higher risk for developing osteoporosis when compared to large boned or obese women and women of African-American descent. You and your doctor can decide what medications or lifestyle changes would best suit you in your quest for better bone health.

Preventing Falls

Falls are the most common cause of injury and injury-related death among older women. They can cause broken bones and hip fractures that may require surgery or end up in total dependence on someone else for care.

The fear of falling can keep aging women from doing the things they want to do in life, which can result in depression, isolation, and loneliness.

Fractures Can Avoided By Preventing Falls:

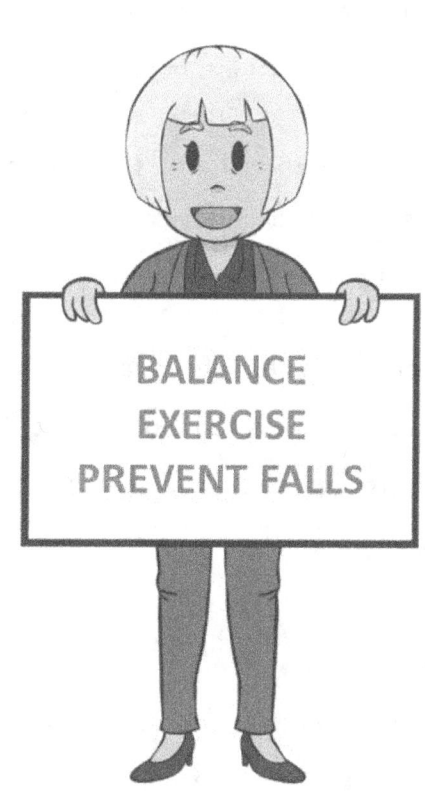

- ✓ Secure your home: get rid of loose rugs in your home, improve lighting, and remove clutter you can trip over.
- ✓ Use a cane, or walker if needed
- ✓ Avoid heavy alcohol intake and try not to use prescription sleeping pills, which can impair your balance.
- ✓ Balance exercises are the best way to ensure that you are strong in this regard and are recommended as part of a regular fitness regimen.
- ✓ Strength training improves muscle mass and gives confidence in being able to tackle everyday activities.
- ✓ Check with your doctor in regards to any medications that can make you dizzy or sleepy.
- ✓ See an eye doctor for an eyesight check every 1 or 2 years.

Brain Health

Women are living longer than ever before, many living into their 80s and 90s. It is therefore more important than ever to make sure these years are filled with fun and exciting experiences, close relationships, better mental health, and an intact memory.

Too many women decide that, just because they are growing older, they will automatically lose their memory and become a burden to their families.

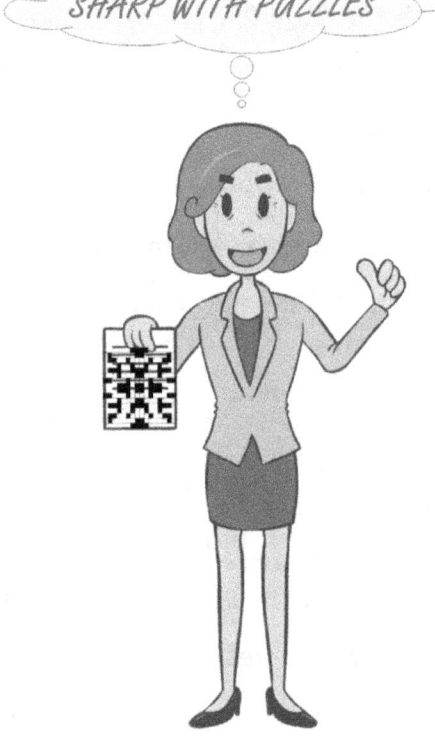

Nothing could be further from the truth. In fact, there are ways you can improve your brain health while aging so that you can be sharp well into your older years.

Improving Brain Health

There are things you can do to better your brain health while dealing with getting older. Women who read books, for example, will retain better memory and will score better on dementia and intelligence scores than women who do not read. You don't have to read volumes of textbooks either. Choose something you enjoy reading and that stimulates your mind so that the synapses between brain cells are maintained and you have a better memory.

Do puzzles, such as Sudoku and crossword puzzles: These will keep your mind sharp and your thinking clearer. Research has shown that women who continue to engage in mentally stimulating activities will have decreased risk of age-related memory loss. There is no reason to lose your memory just because you choose not to exercise your mind.

Engage in physical activity: This can relax you and help you to feel physically stronger. When you are more physically fit, your mind will be clearer and your brain will think better. Physical fitness can be as simple as walking around the block every day, playing golf a couple of times a week, or playing tennis. Swim aerobics is a great group activity that keeps your body and mind as strong as possible.

Continue an active social life as you age: This is a time of loss for some women, who lose friends to cancer or husbands to disease. In spite of having these losses, staying social is very important. You might join a group of women who like the same hobbies you do or that play cards or do physical activity. If, for example, you like gardening, join a group of women (informally or formally) that also like that activity. You can exchange ideas, have fun, and go on outings to keep you physically and mentally challenged. Your brain will deteriorate at a much lesser speed if you continue to "exercise" it.

Avoiding Pitfalls

There are several things you will want to avoid doing if you want to maintain a strong and healthy brain as you age. Some of these include the following:

- **Poor nutrition:** Keep on eating a healthy diet (or adopt one if you haven't been eating healthy). Eating healthy will help you maintain the fuel, nutrients, and vitamins your brain needs to produce all of the necessary brain chemicals used to keep the brain healthy. The brain isn't meant to function on junk food so the more you can eat healthy, the better your brain will function.

- **Remaining sedentary:** Exercise will exercise your brain as well as your mind. When you exercise, you have a greater sense of wellbeing and you can think clearer.

- **Not getting enough sleep:** Research tells us that our memories are solidified and laid down during sleep. This means that if you don't get enough sleep, you can suffer from memory deficits because your memory is lost during sleepless nights. Before long, you can suffer from irritability and concentration difficulties, just because you didn't sleep well for several days in a row.

Your brain health is important. Without it, you can set yourself up for diseases like dementia, depression, and Alzheimer's disease.

Wellness Through Joy And Happiness

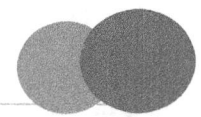

"How old would you be if you didn't know how old you was?" ~ Satchel Paige

As a woman ages, there is an increase in the need for wellness. There is a natural wear and tear on the body that comes with age and there are more diseases that can occur as a woman ages. How does a woman get around some of these natural bodily changes, especially if she has been ignoring her health up until now?

Surprisingly, getting in touch with joy and happiness can improve wellness, including physical and emotional wellness. Because the rates of major depression and other mental disorders tend to increase with age, tying into one's joy and happiness can be a difficult task. Here are some tips to get in touch with your own joy and happiness.

Meditate Daily

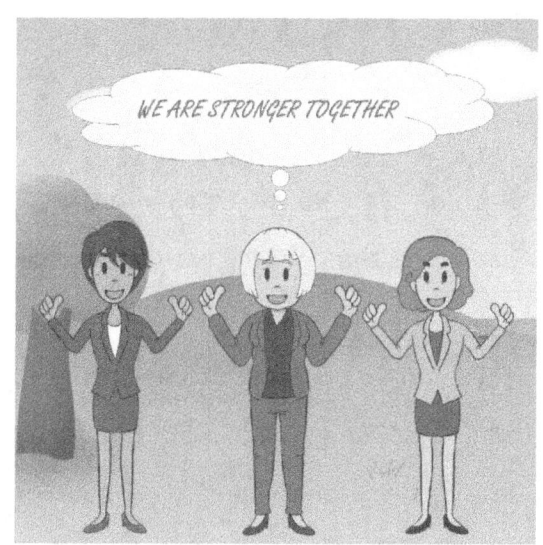

Spend some quiet time focusing on relaxation and breathing. Focus on those things you are thankful for in your life so that you can better enjoy those things that make you happy. Daily meditation has been shown to improve mood and increase happiness. You can meditate for any length of time and at any time of the day for better health and wellness.

Personal Relationships

People feel better when their relationships are in harmony. This includes relationships with siblings, spouses, and children. Don't allow grudges or old angers get in the way of your having a healthy relationship with those you love. It requires open and honest communication with those you love and it may require some forgiveness on your part or on the part of loved ones you've hurt in the past. When old relationship problems are resolved, there will be less room for stress and the health issues that go along with stress.

Stay Social

Older and even middle age years can be a time of isolation, especially if your family has moved out or you have suffered the loss of a spouse through death or divorce. This is not the time to isolate yourself or even to engage in solitary activities. Instead, you can increase the level of joy and happiness in your life by joining social clubs, getting out there to meet more people or to engage in-group sports like golf or even softball. These things can improve your physical health and can bring about a sense of belonging that improves your sense of joy and happiness in your life.

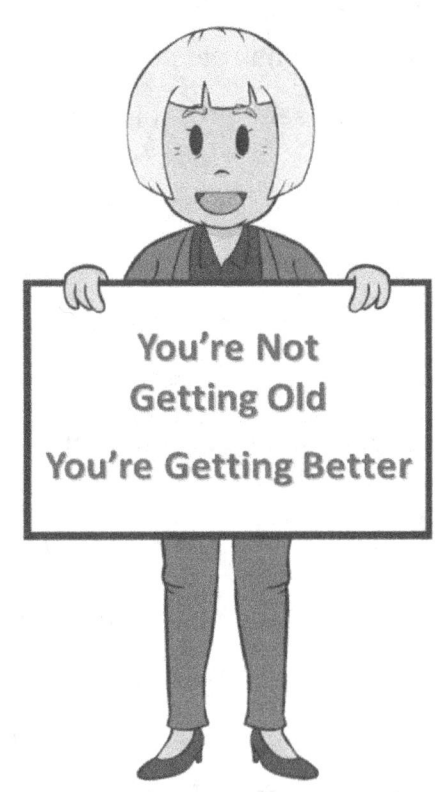

Family

Nothing can help you retain more joy and happiness than playing with your grandchildren, nieces, nephews, or even your own children. These are people that can help you feel young again and can get you out of the doldrums of feeling sorry for yourself and lonely. Grandchildren especially will love you unconditionally and can provide you with endless hours of entertainment that can improve the happiness level in your life.

Having A Purpose

People who live well into their 80s and 90s attest that they have some type of purpose in their life. Be it work, or volunteering, having a purpose promotes wellness, and the desire to stay well and live!

Consequences Of An Unhappy Life

If you isolate yourself or fail to exercise or be social, you run the risk of major depression in your later years, and women suffer depression at a rate of 2 times more than men do. Depression can easily be the result of isolation that can lead to loneliness and disorientation. When you no longer feel a sense of contribution to society, you can feel unhappy and unfulfilled. It takes effort to get out there and be social or even to get some solitary exercise, but the effort is definitely worth it. Those with active social and personal lives enjoy a greater sense of belonging, live longer, and have fewer stress-related diseases such as heart disease, mental illness, stroke, hypertension, and autoimmune diseases.

Those who seek out relationships and social connection, whether it be through group activities or through having a new relationship, will increase the degree of health, wellness and happiness in their lives, making growing older an easier and more pleasurable experience.

"Everyone is always trying to make me younger and I'm tired of that, I just want to be whoever I am right now. Our wrinkles are our medal of the passage of life." ~ Lauren Hutton

Social Interaction To Avoid Depression

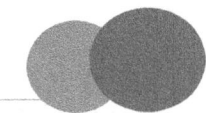

"First you are young; then you are middle-aged; then you are old; then you are wonderful."
~ Lady Diana Cooper

Women over the age of 65 are at a greater risk of depression due to hormonal factors as well as the fact that their male spouses are more likely to die at a younger age, leaving the older woman lonely and feeling socially isolated. Even with solitary hobbies, older women can feel less like they are productive members of society and more like they are a burden on society.

One of the key ways women can avoid late-life depression is to join a social group or at least improve the quality of their social relationships. This can involve social interaction with men or with other women. There are many ways that women can begin to increase their social involvement and therefore improve their wellbeing.

BEING ALONE IS A DOWNER!

- **Join a card club.** You can join a club with likeminded women who play a variety of card games or games like Mahjong. Bridge clubs are everywhere as are clubs that play poker, canasta, or blackjack. These clubs often meet once a week or more often for socializing, drinking, eating, and playing cards at different people's houses. This allows for regular socialization and close friendships.
- **Join a travel club.** If you like to travel and have the means, you can join a travel club of singles and/or couples who create travel plans to destinations all over the world. You can see the world with the same people all the time or you can go with different groups of

people for each vacation. It is much more fun to travel with others and travel clubs offer great opportunities for people of all ages to see exciting and exotic locations.

- **Plan lunch dates.** You can plan lunch dates with another women or several women and try out different restaurants along the way. Lunch or dinner dates can increase conversation (even if it is just about food) and you can meet some lifelong friends this way.

- **Play golf.** While you can play golf by yourself, many people choose to join a golf league and can practice the support with others who like it as well. Some clubs request that you already have a partner, while others allow singletons to join and play golf with a matched pair or with yourself alone with other golfers.

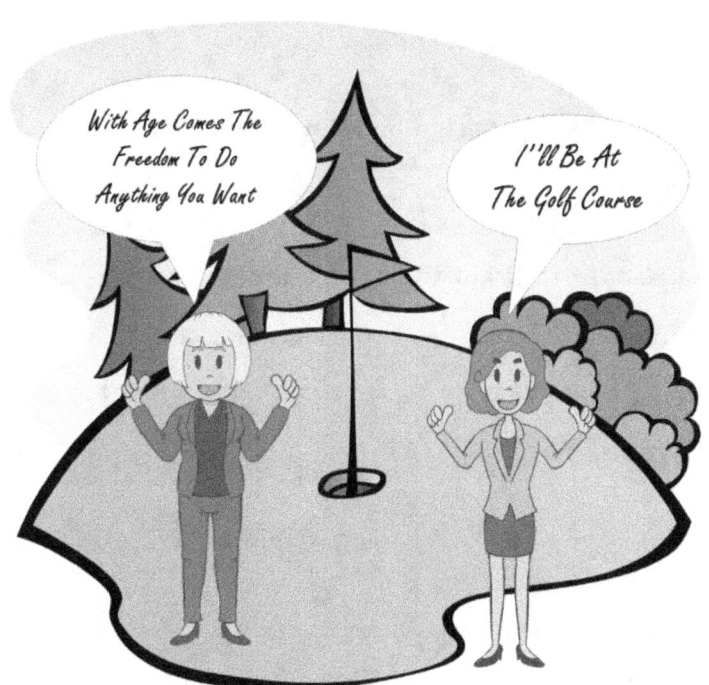

- **Join a tennis or health club.** You can meet people at tennis clubs or at health clubs where they offer tennis lessons, spinning classes, or yoga classes. This can be a year round activity no matter what part of the country you live in and you will meet active people trying to work out, just like you. There are swim aerobic classes that are perfect for older women who want a low impact sport to play in and yet can still meet other people.

- **Join a dating site.** There are dozens of online dating sites, some of which are specifically designed for older men and women. Simply create a personal profile and then look for people that interest you. Through the magic of the computer, you can chat with the person on the web, over the phone or even in person after you decide you want to meet each other.

The importance of socialization in older women cannot be overemphasized enough. Social interaction prolongs mortality and improves the quality of the older woman. It can improve

memory, concentration, and other cognitive strengths. While it isn't always easy to get out there and take the risk to meet more people, being social, especially for an older person, is worth the effort.

Final Thoughts

"Aging is not lost youth but a new stage of opportunity and strength." ~ Betty Friedan

Getting older is a part of life. However, life does not end in the senior years, for many it only beings there.

Thousands of vibrant and energetic seniors are enjoying life as they did in their 30s, 40s, and even their 20s. With age comes wisdom, and wisdom allows us to make better decisions and the self-awareness we have gained throughout life allows us to know what we want and to go and get it.

Embrace your age, and never let a number dictate your quality of life!

Here's To Healthy Aging!